Published By Nicholas Thompson

@ Joseph Landry

Dukan Diet Recipes: Delicious and Nutritious

Meals for for Shedding Weight

All Right RESERVED

ISBN 978-1-990666-98-8

I0558157

TABLE OF CONTENTS

Panfried Lemon Broccoli

Ingredients:

- 3 garlic cloves, chopped

- 23 tbsp. lemon juice

- 1 bunch broccoli

- Salt and pepper to taste

Directions:

1. Wash and break the broccoli into small florets.
2. Pan fry the broccoli and garlic together on high heat for about 12 minutes.
3. Be sure to stir constantly so mixture does not burn. Take pan off heat and cover.

4. Allow to steam for 5 minutes. Season with lemon juice, salt and pepper.

Creamy Chicken Soup

Ingredients:

- 2 garlic cloves

- Pinch of black pepper

- 3 chicken breasts

- ½ lemon for seasoning

- 23 tbsp. oat bran

- ½ large yellow onion

- Pinch of salt

- Pinch of thyme

Directions:

1. Place 2 ½ 3 cups of water into a saucepan to boil.
2. Put all Ingredients: in pan except oats bran.
3. Cook on high heat for 10 minutes, and lower heat to simmer.
4. Continue to cook for 20 minutes. Add oat bran.
5. Blend soup in blender or food processor. Serve hot.

Cream Of Cauliflower Soup

Ingredients:

- 1 head cauliflower, chopped into small pieces

- 2 c. chicken broth

- 2 garlic cloves

- ½ tsp. nutmeg optional

- 1 onion

- 2 tbsp. parsley finely chopped

- ½ tsp. salt

- 2 tbsp. skim milk

- ½ tsp. white pepper

Directions:

1. In a large pot, bring cauliflower, broth and milk to a boil. Add onion and garlic.
2. Cook until tender. Add salt, pepper, nutmeg and parsley before serving.

Ginger Egg Drop Soup

Ingredients:

- 1/8 tsp. ground ginger Salt to taste

- 1 tsp. corn starch

- 1 egg yolk

- 4 cups chicken broth

- 2 tbsp. chives, cleaved

- 2 eggs

Directions:

1. Pour everything except ¾ cup of chicken stock
   into a huge pan. Put away save stock.

2. Add salt, ginger and chives, and bring to a moving bubble. In a bowl, mix together the saved stock and cornstarch until smooth.
3. Set aside. In another bowl, whisk the eggs and egg yolk together utilizing a fork or whisk.
4. Shower egg combination a little at a time, using the fork, into the bubbling broth.
5. Egg should cook immediately.
6. Once all eggs have been dropped, mix the soup until it has reached the ideal consistency.

Baked Dilled Salmon

Ingredients:

- 4 6oz salmon filets

- 4 oz. dry white wine

- 4 new twigs of dill Salt and dark pepper

- Lemon wedges to decorate

Directions:

1. Wash the salmon in cool water and wipe off with a paper towel.
2. Place filets skin side down in a baking dish.
3. Pour wine over salmon and sprinkle with salt and pepper.
4. Put one twig of dill on each filet.

5. Bake the salmon in the broiler for around 2025 minutes, or until it tends to be chipped with fork.

6. Whenever prepared to serve, put filets on serving platter or supper plate and top with a press of new lemon.

Easy Mussel Bake

Ingredients:

- 3.5 lbs. mussels, scoured and flushed

- 1 c. dry white wine

- 3 eggs

- 1 tbsp. nonfat fromage frais, or nonfat cream cheddar

- 2 tbsp. hacked new parsley

- Salt and dark pepper

Directions:

1. Preheat broiler to 450°F.
2. In an enormous, profound pan, place mussels and cover with wine.

11

3. Cover skillet with top and cook on high hotness until mussels start to open.
4. Give the skillet a shake from time to time until they're all open.
5. Discard any mussels that poor person opened.
6. At the point when the mussels are prepared, channel the fluid utilizing a sifter into a bowl.
7. While fluid is still warm, blend in the eggs, fromage frais and parsley with a few salt and dark pepper.
8. Place the mussels in individual ramekins or a soufflé dish, cover with a portion of the messy combination and prepare in the broiler for 10 minutes.
9. Best whenever served immediately!

Leek Soup With Bacon

Ingredients:

- 3 medium turnips, peeled and diced

- 3 rashers low fat bacon, chopped

- 4 liters hot vegetable stock

- 4 rashers low fat bacon, to serve and

- 1 onion, chopped

- 142 ml pot single cream

- 400 grams pack trimmed leeks, sliced.

Directions:

1. Fry the bacons and onion in a nonstick pan, stirring until they become golden. Add in the

leeks and turnips, stir well, turn down the heat and cover the pan. Cook gently for 5 minutes.

2. Pour the stock into the pan, season well and boil. When it does, cover the pan and simmer for 20 minutes to soften the vegetables then remove from heat to cool for a few minutes.

3. Use a food processor to blend the soup until smooth, in batches if necessary, and return to the pan.

4. Pour the cream into the soup and mix well. Season if desired.

5. Enjoy with crumbled bacon.

Salmon Soup Attack

Ingredients:

- Salt for tasting

- 200 grams prawns, shelled

- 200 grams salmon, smoked

- 2 cubes, chicken stock

- Pepper for tasting

- A few spring chives

Directions:

1. After crumbling the chicken stock cubes, boil it in 1 liter of water in a saucepan.

2. While boiling, cut the salmon into thin strips, chop the chives and decorate the prawns separately with the chives.

3. Split the hot stock into soup bowls and throw in the sliced Ingredients: together with pepper.

4. Enjoy immediately with sprinkles chopped chives.

Oat Bran Toast

Ingredients:

- 5 tbsp oat bran

- 3 egg whites

- 3 tbsp zerofat yogurt

Directions:

1. In a bowl, beat the egg whites well – so they become slightly airy.
2. To this, add oat bran and yogurt – stir well.
3. In a nonstick pan, heat a bit of oil and place four round egg rings in it.
4. Divide the egg and oat bran mix into these rings.
5. Once the bottom side is fully cooked, remove them from the rings. Then, proceed to cook the other side.

6. Flatten each piece by applying some pressure count to ten – do not press on it for too long.

7. Once the toast is ready, grill – do so till both sides are brown. This can be eaten hot or cold.

Scrambled Eggs With Herbs

Ingredients:

- 2 tbsp skimmed milk

- 3 eggs

- 2 scallions, finely sliced

- ¼ tbsp coriander, chopped

- ¼ tbsp fresh parsley, chopped

- ¼ tbsp fresh chives, chopped

Directions:

1. In a bowl, mix the skimmed milk, eggs, scallions and herbs. Beat the mixture till the yolks are well mixed.

2. Place it in the microwave that is on full power – for about 45 seconds.
3. Remove it from the microwave – stir to mix again. Place it in the microwave for 15 seconds.
4. Repeat this till the eggs achieve the consistency you think is perfect.

Zucchini Lasagna

Ingredients:

- 7 oz. ground beef, lean

- 3 ½ oz. mozzarella cheese, light

- 1 tbsp. tomato extract, pure

- ½ onion, medium

- 3 ½ oz. turkey breast, smoked

- Ground pepper

- 1 garlic clove

- Oregano, chives, parsley, kosher salt and

- 2 lengthwisesliced zucchinis, medium

- 2 peeled, deseeded tomatoes, ripe, large

Directions:

1. Grill each side of sliced zucchinis in nonstick pan. Set aside.
2. Sauté onion and garlic in pan on low heat.
3. Add kosher salt, ground pepper and beef. Cook on low.
4. Pour 1 ¾ oz. of filtered water in food processor.
5. Add chives, parsley and tomatoes diced. Combine till smooth.
6. Add sauce to beef. Add tomato extract. Boil mixture for 1215 minutes.
7. Add some sauce to baking dish/pizza form for oven cooking.
8. Form layers using zucchini, then turkey breast, then cheese and sauce.
9. Repeat layers two times. Top with cheese and oregano.

10. Place in oven for 2025 minutes. Then turn
    oven to off. Allow lasagna to sit for 1215
    minutes. Serve.

Chicken Marsala

Ingredients:

- 1/3 of 1 small onion, red

- 2 tbsp. milk, skim

- 1 tbsp. curry powder

- 3 tbsp. garam masala Middle Eastern spice mix

- 1 handful mushrooms

- 1 tbsp. garlic powder

- 1 chicken breast

Directions:

1. Butterflycut chicken thinly, so it cooks quicker. Add curry powder and garlic salt on each side of chicken.
2. Use oven or grill to cook chicken till both sides are brown.
3. As chicken cooks, slice mushrooms and onions into pieces of 1/2inch or so. Add to sauté pan.
4. As the mushrooms start shrinking, add milk. Turn heat down. Allow to simmer for about five more minutes.
5. Place chicken on plates and spread the onion and mushroom mixture over the top. Serve.

Spinach Pie

Ingredients:

- 2 beaten eggs, large

- 2 1/2 ounces of without fat cheddar, feta

- 8 3/4 oz. of ricotta cheddar, fatfree

- 8 3/4 oz. of cleaved spinach, frozen

- 1/2 tsp. of nutmeg, ground

- 1 modest bunch of basil leaves, chopped

- 1 modest bunch of tomatoes, cherry

- Salt, kosher

- Pepper, dark, ground

Directions:

1. Preheat stove to 325F.
2. Thaw the spinach in your microwave. Press it and channel water.
3. Mix ricotta cheddar with genuine salt, ground pepper, basil, nutmeg, spinach and eggs in huge estimated bowl. Join well.
4. Spray baking dish with oil. Pour in spinach combination. Spread till even.
5. Garnish with divided cherry tomatoes.
6. Sprinkle with cheddar around tomatoes.
7. Place dish in broiler. Cook for 35 to 40 minutes, until combination has set well.
8. During last 5 cooking minutes, place dish under barbecue to brown tomatoes and cheddar.
9. Serve warm. It can likewise be served cold, on the off chance that you prefer.

General Tso's Chicken

Ingredients:

- 1/3 cup of corn starch

- Nonstick spray

- 3 minced cuts of ginger, peeled

- 1 minced garlic clove

- 4 or 5 decultivated, washed, dried chilies, red

- 2 stalks of green onion, just the white part, cut small

- 10 ounces of reduced down cut chicken bosom or thigh meat, skinless, boneless

- 1/2 tbsp. of wine, Shaoxing

- 1 squeeze salt, kosher

- Tso sauce, bottled

Directions:

1. Marinate chicken meat in fit salt and Shaoxing wine for 12 to 15 minutes.
2. Generously cover chicken with corn starch. Heat nonstick container.
3. Fry chicken till it turns lighter brown. Eliminate chicken utilizing sifter.
4. Channel off abundance fat onto paper towels.
5. Heat up skillet with 1 1/2 tbsp. of nonstick shower.
6. Add chilies, ginger and garlic into skillet.
7. Pan sear till you can undoubtedly smell the chilies' aroma.
8. Pour tso sauce into skillet. Whenever it thickens and bubbles, add chicken.

9. Consolidate by blending with sauce. Add green onions. Mix a few times. Serve hot in individual dishes.

Rosemary Roasted Turkey

Ingredients:

- ¾ cup olive oil

- 3 tablespoons minced garlic

- 2 tablespoons chopped fresh rosemary

- 1 tablespoon chopped fresh basil

- 1 tablespoon Italian seasoning

- 1 teaspoon ground black pepper

- salt to taste

- 1 12 pound whole turkey

Directions:

1. Preheat oven to 325 degrees F 165 degrees C.

2. In a small bowl, mix the olive oil, garlic, rosemary, basil, Italian seasoning, black pepper and salt. Set aside.

3. Wash the turkey inside and out pat dry. Remove any large fat deposits. Loosen the skin from the breast.

4. This is done by slowly working your fingers between the breast and the skin.

5. Work it loose to the end of the drumstick, being careful not to tear the skin.

6. Using your hand, spread a generous amount of the rosemary mixture under the breast skin and down the thigh and leg.

7. Rub the remainder of the rosemary mixture over the outside of the breast.

8. Use toothpicks to seal skin over any exposed breast meat.

9. Place the turkey on a rack in a roasting pan.

10. Add about 1/4 inch of water to the bottom of the pan.
11. Roast in the preheated oven 3 to 4 hours, or until the internal temperature of the bird reaches 180 degrees F 80 degrees C.

Coriander Sole

Ingredients:

- 3 tablespoons white wine tolerated

- 2 sprigs of fresh coriander

- 2 fillets of sole

- ½ lemon

- Salt and pepper

Directions:

1. Marinate 2 fillets of sole for 1 2 hours in a mixture of lemon juice and white wine in equal parts, seasoned with fresh coriander, salt and pepper.
2. Brown in a nonstick pan with the marinade.
3. Sprinkle with coriander before serving.

Baked Bass

Ingredients:

- 2 tomatoes, cut in ½

- 1 lemon, cut into slices

- A handful of fresh parsley, finely chopped 1 clove of garlic, crushed through a garlic press

- 2 fresh bass fish fillets

- 2 onions, peeled and sliced into strips

- Salt and pepper

Directions:

1. Preheat the oven to 375 F.

2. Lay the onions onto an oven proof baking dish.
3. Lay the bass fillets on top of the onions, and surround with the cut tomatoes.
4. Lay the lemon slices over the fillets with any remaining around the fish with the tomatoes.
5. Sprinkle the tomatoes with the herbs and crushed garlic, and season with salt and pepper.
6. Bake for 2030 minutes or until the meat has turned white, checking close to the end time to ensure the fish does not overcook.

Suitable Protein Patty Soup

Ingredients:

- 2 tablespoon bran, oat, easily soluble flakes

- 50 ml milk, 1.5%

- 1 pinch s salt

- 3 drops olive oil

- 10 g broth, instant

- 1 liter water

- 2 large egg s

Directions:

1. Bring the water and stock powder to the boil together.

2. Dissolve the oat bran in the milk in a container. Add the eggs and whisk everything together. Add the salt.

3. Let a pan rubbed with a few drops of oil add 34 drops of oil to the pan and rub the whole thing with a paper towel warm up. Slowly cook the Flädle mixture in the pan it should ideally be golden brown on both sides.

4. Turning it around is a bit difficult, but Flädle naturally forgives small mistakes, they will be cut up anyway.

5. Let the pancake cool briefly and then cut into strips the length of the strips can be adjusted to personal preference. Add the pancakes to the soup and enjoy.

6. Tip for turning: I use two dough scrapers at the same time.

7. Because this type of pancake loves to break. The best chance of turning it whole or at least in half is with several scrapers.

8. Info: for the sake of simplicity, I use soup powder but in homeopathic dilution because of the fat and salt.

9. For Dukan fans: the recipe is also suitable for the attack phase.

10. You just have to pay attention to the fat and salt because of the broth but the soup is the most important thing.

11. For Dukan newbies: the diet is about not eating any carbohydrates after an initial phase, they are allowed again every other day in the form of vegetables, but of course no potatoes or the like the diet is therefore only for real meat and suitable for yoghurt lovers.

Endive And Caviar Salad

Ingredients:

- 1 tablespoon lumpfish or salmon roe

- 1 tablespoon white wine vinegar

- 2 heads of endive

- ¼ cup fatfree sour cream

Directions:

1. Slice the endive down the middle and then again across.
2. Place the leaves into a salad bowl.
3. For the dressing: mix the sour cream, caviar, and vinegar.
4. Toss the dressing with the endives.

Easy Seafood Stirfry

Ingredients:

- 1 teaspoon olive oil, divided tolerated

- ½ pound bay scallops or halved sea scallops

- ¼ pound medium raw shrimp, peeled and deveined 2 cloves of garlic, minced

- 2 cups of green beans

- ¼ cup of thinly sliced green onions

- "2 packs of Dukan Diet Shirataki rice

- 1 ounce of dried shiitake mushrooms or 1.5 cups of fresh mushrooms

- ½ cup of fatfree, low sodium chicken broth

- 1 tablespoon low sodium soy sauce

- 4.5 teaspoons of cornstarch tolerated

Directions:

1. Prepare Shirataki rice according to package instructions and set aside.
2. Place mushrooms in small bowl cover with boiling water.
3. Soak 20 minutes to soften. Drain squeeze out excess water. Discard stems slice caps.
4. Blend broth and soy sauce into cornstarch in another small bowl until smooth set aside.
5. Heat ½ teaspoon oil in wok or skillet over medium heat. Add scallops,
6. shrimp and garlic stirfry 3 minutes or until seafood is opaque. Remove and reserve.
7. Add remaining ½ teaspoon oil to wok.
8. Add mushrooms and green beans stirfry 3 minutes or until green beans are crisptender.

9. Stir broth mixture add to wok. Cook and stir 2 minutes or until sauce boils and thickens.

10. Return seafood and any accumulated juices to wok cook and stir until heated through. Sprinkle with green onions.

11. Plate with the Shirataki rice.

Chicken With Lemons

Ingredients:

- 2 garlic cloves, finely chopped

- 1 teaspoon peeled and finely chopped fresh ginger

- 1 pound boneless, skinless chicken breasts, cut into 1inch cubes

- Grated zest and juice of 2 lemons

- 2 tablespoons lowsodium soy sauce

- ⅛ teaspoon vegetable oil

- 1 onion, finely chopped

- 1 bouquet garni make your own by tying together 6 sprigs of fresh parsley, 3 sprigs of fresh thyme, and 3 dried bay leaves

- A pinch of ground cinnamon

- A pinch of ground ginger

- Salt and freshly ground black pepper

Directions:

1. Heat a deep nonstick skillet over medium heat.
2. Add the oil and wipe out any excess with a paper towel.
3. Add the onion, garlic, and fresh ginger and cook for 3 to 4 minutes, or until browned.
4. Increase the heat to high, add the chicken, and sauté for 2 minutes, stirring constantly.
5. Add the lemon zest, lemon juice, soy sauce, $\frac{2}{3}$ cup of water, and the bouquet garni,

cinnamon, and ground ginger. Add salt and pepper to taste. Reduce the heat to a gentle simmer, cover, and cook for 20 minutes.

6. Add the onion and cook until brown, about 3 minutes.

7. Add the chili, curry powder, cinnamon, and clove.

8. Add salt and pepper to taste, and cook for another 2 minutes, stirring continuously.

9. Add the eggplant, tomatoes, and stock.

10. Simmer for 40 minutes with the saucepan half covered. In a blender, process the soup until smooth, about 30 seconds.

11. Reheat the soup before serving, adjusting the salt and pepper to taste.

Baked Eggs With Tomato Basil Sauce

Ingredients:

- A pinch of ground nutmeg

- Salt and freshly ground black pepper

- ⅛ teaspoon vegetable oil

- 6 tomatoes, stems and seeds removed, diced

- 4 eggs

- ¾ cup fatfree milk

- 3 basil leaves

Directions:

1. Preheat oven to 350°F.

2. In a medium bowl, beat the eggs with the milk, nutmeg, and salt and pepper to taste.

3. Coat two 1cup ramekins with the oil and wipe out any excess with a paper towel. Fill with the egg mixture.

4. Place the ramekins in a bigger baking dish and fill the baking dish halfway with cold water. Bake for 40 minutes.

5. While the egg mixture is baking, place the tomatoes, basil, and salt and pepper to taste in a medium pot and cook over medium heat, stirring occasionally until it becomes a thick sauce, about 20 minutes.

6. Turn the baked eggs out of the ramekins and pour the sauce over them. Serve hot.

Chicken Breasts Morocco

Ingredients:

- 2 teaspoons minced garlic

- 2 tablespoons lemon juice

- ¼ teaspoon red pepper flakes, optional if you like it spicy!

- 4 boneless, skinless chicken breasts

- 2 tablespoons Moroccan Spice Mix see below for simple recipe

- 2 tablespoons Dijon mustard

Directions:

1. Combine first 5 Ingredients: in large bowl and mix well to combine.

2. Add chicken breasts and turn to coat with the spice mixture.
3. Cover the bowl with transparent cling wrap and allow to marinate for at least 2 hours or overnight.
4. The longer you marinate, the more intense the flavor will be.
5. When you are ready to cook, discard the marinade.
6. Broil or grill the chicken breasts for 57 minutes on each side, or until juices run clear when the breast is pricked with a fork.

Beef Kebabs

Ingredients:

- 2 tablespoons Dijon mustard

- Dash of olive oil

- ¼ cup fresh lemon juice

- ¼ teaspoon dried thyme

- 1 bay leaf

- 16 oz beef fillet

- 1 tablespoon apple cider vinegar

- ¼ cup low sodium soy sauce

Directions:

1. Cut the meat into 1inch cubes.
2. Mix all the other Ingredients: in a large bowl.
3. Place the meat in the marinade, cover with transparent cling wrap and refrigerate for at least 2 hours or overnight.
4. The longer it marinates, the more intense the flavor. When ready to cook, discard the marinade.
5. Assemble the beef onto skewers. If using wooden skewers, be sure to soak them for at least 30 minutes to avoid burning.
6. Grill or broil the kebabs until the meat is done according to your own preference.

Rosemary Beef Burgers

Ingredients:

For burger

- Chopped fresh rosemary 2 tbsp

- Lean beef 450 gm, minced

- 1 whole egg

- Nutmeg 1 tsp

- Oat bran 3 tbsp

- Freshly ground black pepper

For dip

- Greek yogurt 250 gm

- Smoked paprika 1 tsp

- Dried dill 2 tsp

Directions:

1. For dip, blend all the Ingredients: together in a bowl.
2. Cover and place in the refrigerator to chill.
3. For burger, combine all the Ingredients: in a food processor and process until smooth and then make burgers from the batter by molding.
4. Place the griddle pan few minutes over high heat and then cook burgers on it until brown.
5. Serve and enjoy the delicious recipe.

Mini Burgers

Ingredients:

- 1 green chili, chopped [optional]

- Chicken breast 500 gm, minced

- 1 egg

- 2 small garlic cloves, chopped

- Oat bran 2 tbsp

- Cajun spice mix 1 tbsp

Directions:

1. Blend chicken breast along with the rest of the Ingredients: in a blender until form smooth batter.

2. Shape the mixture and form burgers by using your hands.

3. Heat the griddle pan for few minutes over high heat.

4. Arrange burgers on the pan and cook until done.

5. Serve with Greek yogurt.

Steak Pizzaiola

Ingredients:

- Tomato paste 2 tbsp

- 2 garlic cloves, sliced

- Lean beef

- A handful of chopped flat leaf parsley

- Cooking spray

Directions:

1. Grease the frying pan with a cooking spray and add beef.
2. Dilute the tomato paste by adding few tablespoons of water and daub the paste around the meat.

3. Add garlic and half of the chopped parsley and cook over medium high heat for about 15 minutes until done.
4. If the tomato sauce gets thick during the cooking process then add a little hot water.
5. Flavor the steak with black pepper and splash with chopped parsley while serving.

Patties With A Twist

Ingredients:

- ¼ teaspoon dried marjoram

- 1 tablespoon brown sugar

- 1/8 teaspoon crushed red pepper flakes

- 1 pinch ground cloves

- 2 pounds ground pork

- 2 teaspoons dried sage

- 2 teaspoons salt

- 1 teaspoon ground black pepper

Directions:

1. Set aside ground pork in a big bowl. In a smaller bowl, add all spices, and mix well.

2. Pour over the premixed spices over the meat. Thoroughly blend the meat with the spices to even out the taste, using your bare, clean hands.

3. After mixing, form patties that are not too thick or too thin.

4. Cook the patties in preheated oil in a frying pan, until the meat is completely cooked.

Piquant Sausage And Ground Turkey Meatballs

Ingredients:

- 1 20 ounce package spicy Italian ground turkey

- 3 eggs

- ¼ onion, minced

- 1 20 ounce package bulk spicy Italian turkey sausage

- ¼ teaspoon ground black pepper

Directions:

1. Prior to Directions: of the meatball mixture, preheat the oven to 350 degrees F 175 degrees C.

2. Add all Ingredients: into a mixing bowl, and ensure even distribution of the onion, pepper, and egg amongst the sausage and ground turkey.

3. You may also try adding the sausage and ground turkey first, and then slowly adding other Ingredients:. Make rolls of about 1 ½ inch balls.

4. Line balls along a baking sheet. Bake for 1820 minutes, or until juice comes out of each ball.

Oilfree Chocolate Muffins | Plantbased Desserts

Ingredients:

- 6 tablespoons water

- 2 tablespoons ground flax seed heaping tablespoons

- 1 1/2 teaspoons baking powder

- 1 teaspoon arrowroot powder

- 1 teaspoon vanilla extract

- 1/4 teaspoon salt

- 15 ounces black beans can, without the liquid, or 1 3/4 cups cooked

- 3/4 cup cacao powder

- 1/2 cup coconut palm sugar heaping cup

- 1 banana small or 1/2 large

- 1/4 cup unsweetened applesauce

Directions:

1. Preheat oven to 350.
2. Puree all ingredients until smooth – the consistency should be less thick than frosting but not runny.
3. Spoon equal quantity of the mixture into baking cup liners in a 12 cup standard size muffin tin – cups should be about half full.
4. Bake 30 minutes at 350 degrees – muffin tops should be dry, slightly raised and cracked.
5. Let cool for at least 30 minutes then enjoy!

Oilfree Blueberry Scones Glutenfree

Ingredients:

- 2 tablespoons chia seeds

- 1/2 teaspoon salt optional

- 1/4 cup unsweetened plant milk

- 3 tablespoons maple syrup

- 1 tablespoon lemon juice

- 1 teaspoon pure vanilla extract

- 1 cup blueberries fresh or frozen

- Powdered Sugar Drizzle optional

- 1/2 cup Powdered sugar loosely packe

- 1 tablespoon plant milk

- 1 tablespoon flax meal

- 2 tablespoons water

- 1 1/4 cups oat flour

- 1 1/4 cups blanched almond flour tightly packed

- 1 tablespoon baking powder

Directions:

1. Preheat oven to 400°F. Line a baking sheet with parchment paper.
2. Mix the flax meal with the water and set aside.
3. Whisk oat flour, almond flour, baking powder, chia seeds, and salt in a bowl.

4. Combine flax mixture with soymilk, maple syrup, lemon juice, and vanilla and add to the dry ingredients.

5. Mix carefully until just combined. The dough is thick and sticky. You might need to use your hands to pull it together. Add a tablespoon or more plant milk if it's too dry.

6. Very gently fold in the blueberries.

7. On a lightly floured surface, shape the scone mixture into a 7" circle.

8. Place onto the baking sheet, cut into 8 wedges, and gently pull them apart so there's at least an inch between them. **To make round scones, see the instructions in the recipe notes below.

9. Bake on the middle rack for 1520 minutes until lightly golden brown. Check at 15 minutes to see if they're golden brown yet as each oven is different.

10. To top with a powdered sugar drizzle mix 1/2 cup loosely packed powdered sugar with 1 tablespoon plant milk and mix until smooth. Drizzle across each scone.

11. If you have leftovers, refrigerate in an airtight container for about 7 days or frozen up to 3 months.

Ham And Vegetable Soup

Ingredients:

- 1 large yellow onion

- 1 can tomatoes

- 3 cloves garlic, minced

- 1 tbsp. fatfree quark

- 3 slices turkey ham

- ½ c. fresh basil, coarsely chopped

- About 1 ¾ c. vegetable stock

Directions:

1. Heat a saucepan, and add a little bit of water.

2. Add garlic and onions and sauté for few minutes.
3. Add canned tomatoes and stir, crushing the tomatoes with spoon.
4. Add vegetable stock. Stir and add sliced ham and basil.
5. Cook on low heat for around 40 minutes. Serve topped with quark and fresh basil.

Egg And Tomato Muffins

Ingredients:

- ½ tsp. garlic powder

- ½ onion

- Handful of parsley

- 1 green pepper

- 2 eggs

- 1 small tomato

Directions:

1. Preheat oven to 350°F.
2. Combine Ingredients: with hand mixer or blender.

3. Place mixture in nonstick cupcake tray. Cook for 15 minutes.
4. Tastes great topped with fatfree cream cheese!

Smooth And Creamy Cauliflower Mash

Ingredients:

- Butter flavoring optional

- 3 tbsp. fatfree cream cheese

- 12 garlic cloves, peeled

- 1 whole cauliflower

- Salt and pepper to taste

Directions:

1. Break the cauliflower into pieces using hands.
2. Place pieces in steamer with garlic cloves. Steam until vegetables very tender 3035 minutes.

3. Using a piece of cheesecloth, squeeze as much moisture from the cauliflower as you can. The drier you can get it, the better.
4. Whip the cauliflower, garlic, cream cheese, butter flavoring, salt and pepper until smooth.
5. Serve similarly to a mashed potato.

Delicious Turkey Meatballs

Ingredients:

- 1 lb lean ground turkey

- 1 enormous onion, coarsely ground

- 1 garlic clove, finely slashed

- 1 tsp. oregano

- 1 tsp. dried basil

- 1 egg

- Salt and dark pepper

- Plain fat free yogurt

Directions:

1. Combine fixings in a huge bowl aside from yogurt.
2. Utilize your hands to combine as one, being certain all fixings are circulated well.
3. Fry meatballs in a nonstick skillet until cooked.
4. Finish in grill or hot stove. Present with plain yogurt.

Salmon N' Eggs

Ingredients:

- ¾ c. skimmed milk

- 2 tbsp. without fat fromage frais or nonfat cream cheddar

- 5 chive stalks, chopped

- 10 Eggs

- Salt and pepper Garlic powder

- 5oz smoked salmon, cut into meager pieces

Directions:

1. Beat eggs together in a huge bowl and season daintily with the salt, dark pepper and garlic powder.

2. Warm skim milk in an enormous sauce container.

3. Pour in the beaten eggs and cook over a delicate hotness.

4. Make certain to continually mix so the eggs don't adhere to the skillet.

5. Once cooked to wanted consistency, eliminate from hotness and mix in the salmon and fromage frais.

6. Serve right away. For a hint of excellence and flavor, design with a couple of chives and parsley.

Filling Bacon And Cheese Stuffed Chicken

Ingredients:

- 2 boneless, skinless chicken breasts

- 4 piling tbsp. Quark or mix of 9 sections lowfat ricotta and 1 section without fat harsh cream

- Handful of hacked chives

- 4 cuts turkey bacon

- Freshly ground dark pepper

Directions:

1. Preheat broiler to 400°F.
2. Take chicken filets and cut 2 little pockets into side of the chicken for filling.

3. Season each side of chicken with salt and pepper and put away. In a little bowl, consolidate the Quark and the cleaved chives.
4. Spoon half of the blend into the pocket one of the chicken bosom filets, and the other half into the subsequent bosom.
5. Wrap every chicken bosom with 2 cuts of turkey bacon.
6. The bacon will give added flavor and assist with holding a portion of the chicken' s juices.
7. Place the stuffed chicken onto a baking sheet, and prepare for 25 and 30 minutes, or until the chicken is cooked and squeezes run clear.
8. For the most ideal flavor and firm bacon!, serve immediately.

Oat Bran Galette

Ingredients:

- 2 egg whites

- 3 tablespoons 0% fat Greek yogurt and

- 3 tablespoons oat bran.

Directions:

1. Whisk together the Ingredients: in a bowl until you arrive at a smooth liquid batter. If it seems too thick, add more yogurt to thin out.
2. Grease the bottom of a nonstick pan lightly and pour in half of the batter, cooking on medium heat until both sides turn golden brown.
3. Repeat the process for the remaining half of the batter.

Dukanoffe Frap Attack

Ingredients:

- 16 ice cubes and

- 4 teaspoons aspartame.

- 1 cup skimmed milk straight from the fridge

- 1 cup strong black coffee or espresso, cold

Directions:

1. Blend the milk, coffee and sweetener in a blender until they become a nice, foamy mixture.
2. Blend the ice in until broken into small chunks.
3. After stirring well, pour into 2 tall glasses and enjoy!

Poultry Bacon Egg Sandwich

Ingredients:

- 8 lowfat turkey bacon rashers

- A pinch of dried dill and

- Black pepper, freshly ground.

- 2 eggs

- 2 oat bran galettes, flavored with your favorite herbs

Directions:

1. While preheating your grill to 356 degrees F, prepare 2 oat bran galettes using the first recipe but add more flavor by using fresh or dried herbs on the batter prior to cooking.

2. Once the galettes are done, place each on a plate to set aside.

3. Use tin foil to line a baking tray on which you'll place the turkey bacon rashers for grilling.

4. Put the baking tray under the grill to cook for 10 to 15 minutes.

5. When the bacon rashers are near cooked, start to poach the eggs either manually using the swirl Directions: or us a Poach pod, a.k.a. a silicone egg poacher. Sprinkle each egg with a pinch of dried dill prior to poaching.

6. Once the bacons are done, place them on top of the oat bran galettes, topped by a poached egg each.

7. Use freshly ground black pepper to season and enjoy!

Oat Bran Muffins

Ingredients:

- ¼ cup skimmed milk

- 3 eggs

- 6 tablespoons fat free natural yogurt and

- Vanilla extract, to taste.

- 1 ½ cups oat bran

- 1 cup baking Splenda

- 1 teaspoon baking powder

Directions:

1. After mixing all the Ingredients: well, let them sit for about 20 minutes.

2. While waiting, spray some cooking oil to line a nonstick muffin tin.
3. Fill the tin/s with the mixture and bake at 350 degrees F until done.

Zesty Lemon Pancakes

Ingredients:

- 2 tbsp oat bran

- 8 tbsp fatfree yogurt

- 4 tbsp sweetener

- 2 eggs

- 2 egg whites

- Zest of a lemon

Directions:

1. In a bowl, beat the egg whites and eggs together.
2. To this, add oat bran, yogurt, sweetener and lemon zest – make sure you stir well.

3. In a nonstick pan, heat a few drops of oil – make sure it spreads to all corners of the pan.

4. Place some of the pancake batter onto the pan. Cook on medium heat, till bubbles form on the pancake.

5. Then, turn the pancake and continue letting it cook – till the pancake becomes brown in color.

6. Repeat the process till all of the batter has been used.

Breakfast Frittata

Ingredients:

- 1 ½ tomatoes, diced and deseeded

- 1 ½ cups mushrooms, thinly sliced

- ¾ onion, diced

- 3 tbsp fresh chives, chopped

- 9 eggs

- 3 tbsp vegetable stock

- Sea salt, according to taste

- Black pepper, ground, according to taste

Directions:

1. Use ½ tbsp of the stock to sauté the onion on medium heat, till the onion becomes soft.
2. Next, add another ½ tbsp of the stock, and add the mushrooms to it.
3. Cook again for around 34 minutes, till fully cooked.
4. Add the rest of the stock, and the tomato and cook some more.
5. In a bowl, beat the eggs together. Next, add the chives and make sure the eggs are well seasoned.
6. Pour the egg mixture on the pan – cook on low heat.
7. Cover and continue to cook till the eggs become firm.
8. Cut into pieces according to a chosen size then serve.

Piri Piri Chicken

Ingredients:

- 1 tsp chili flakes, crushed

- ½ tsp paprika

- ½ tsp oregano

- 2 tbsp cider vinegar

- ½ tsp lemon juice

- ½ tsp lime juice

- Sea salt, according to taste

- 2 chicken breast fillets, skinless

- 1 clove of garlic, finely chopped

- Black pepper, ground, according to taste

- Fatfree yogurt, according to taste

Directions:

1. In a bowl, prepare a marinade by mixing the garlic, chili flakes, paprika, oregano, cider vinegar and lemon juice together.
2. Place each piece of chicken in the marinade and coat the fillet thoroughly.
3. Cover this bowl with cling wrap and place it in the refrigerator overnight.
4. The next day, remove the chicken from the bowl and season with salt and pepper according to taste.
5. Grill on medium heat, till the fillets are thoroughly cooked.
6. Serve along with fatfree yogurt, after adding the lime juice to it.

Spinach Pie

Ingredients:

- Salt, kosher

- 8 ¾ oz. ricotta cheese, fatfree

- 2 ½ oz. fatfree cheese, feta

- 8 ¾ oz. chopped spinach, frozen

- ½ tsp. nutmeg, ground

- 1 handful basil leaves, chopped

- Black pepper, ground

- 1 handful tomatoes, cherry

- 2 beaten eggs, large

Directions:

1. Preheat oven to 325F.

2. Thaw the spinach in your microwave oven. Squeeze it and drain water.

3. Mix ricotta cheese with kosher salt, ground pepper, basil, nutmeg, spinach and eggs in large sized bowl. Combine well.

4. Spray baking dish with oil. Pour in spinach mixture. Spread till even.

5. Garnish with halved cherry tomatoes. Sprinkle with cheese around tomatoes.

6. Place dish in oven. Cook for 35 to 40 minutes, until mixture has set well.

7. During last 5 cooking minutes, place dish under grill to brown tomatoes and cheese.

8. Serve warm. It can also be served cold if you prefer.

Basil Thai Chicken

Ingredients:

- 2 slivered lime leaves, kaffir

- 3 tsp. soy sauce, sweet, black

- 6 chopped, pounded bird Thai chilies

- 2 eggs, large

- ½ lb. cubed chicken, boneless

- 2 diced shallots

- 4 minced garlic cloves

- 1 pinch pepper, white

- Large bunch stemremoved Thai basil, sweet

- 1 tbsp. fish sauce, Thai

- Nonstick spray

- 2 tsp. Splenda

Directions:

1. Spray heated skillet, then add shallots and garlic.
2. Stir fry them till they are aromatic.
3. Add chicken meat. Stir fry quickly. Break chicken meat into small sized lumps.
4. When chicken has changed color, add chilies and seasonings. Continue stirfrying.
5. Add basil leaves. Stir a few times till basil leaves wilt and you smell their exotic fragrance.
6. Sprinkle 2 dashes of white pepper powder in mixture.
7. Stir one last time. Transfer to dishes. Serve promptly.

Roasted Brussels Sprouts

Ingredients:

- 2 tbsp. vinegar, balsamic

- 2 tsp. honey, organic

- 3 tbsp. oil, olive

- 1 ½ lb. Brussels sprouts, frozen

- ¼ tsp. pepper, black

- ½ tsp. salt, kosher

Directions:

1. Preheat the oven to 425F. Line a large sized cookie sheet with baking paper.
2. Trim ends from Brussels sprouts. Peel off any wilted leaves and toss them.

3. Arrange the Brussels sprouts on a cookie sheet. Use oil to drizzle.

4. Season using kosher salt and ground pepper.

5. Toss and coat the sprouts evenly. Spread them out into one layer with no pieces overlapping.

6. Roast the Brussels sprouts for 1520 minutes, till the edges are caramelized. Remove them from the oven.

7. Whisk vinegar and honey together in a small sized bowl.

8. Pour this mixture over the roasted Brussels sprouts. Evenly coat by tossing and serve promptly.

Roasted Brussels Sprouts

Ingredients:

- 3 tbsp. of oil, olive

- 1/2 tsp. of salt, kosher

- 1/4 tsp. of pepper, black

- 2 tbsp. of vinegar, balsamic

- 1 1/2 pounds of Brussels sprouts, frozen or fresh

- 2 tsp. of honey, organic

Directions:

1. Preheat the stove to 425F.

2. Line huge estimated treat sheet with baking paper.
3. Trim closures from Brussels sprouts. Strip off any withered leaves and throw them.
4. Arrange the Brussels sprouts on treat sheet. Use oil to sprinkle.
5. Season utilizing fit salt and ground pepper.
6. Throw and coat the fledglings equitably.
7. Spread them out into one layer without any pieces overlapping.
8. Roast the Brussels sprouts for 1520 minutes, till the edges are caramelized. Eliminate them from the oven.
9. Whisk vinegar and honey together in little measured bowl.
10. Pour this combination over the simmered Brussels sprouts.
11. Equitably coat by throwing and serve promptly.

Sticky Asian Chicken

Ingredients:

- 3 tbsp. of soy sauce, low sodium

- 1 tsp. of Splenda

- 2 tsp. of stew paste

- 8 chicken strips or thighs, boneless, skinless

- 3 tbsp. of vinegar, balsamic

Directions:

1. Brown each side of chicken pieces in skillet preshowered with nonstick splash.
2. Thighs will typically require around five minutes for every side, and tenders will frequently be done quickly per side.
3. Combine rest of fixings in sauce skillet.

4. Bring to bubble. Stew for five minutes. Combination ought to have thickened.

5. After chicken is sautéed, add sauce to skillet.

6. Cook for around five to 10 minutes for chicken thighs or five to seven minutes for chicken fingers. Serve.

Whole chicken slow cooker

Ingredients:

- 4 teaspoons salt, or to taste

- 2 teaspoons paprika

- 1 teaspoon cayenne pepper

- 1 teaspoon onion powder

- 1 teaspoon ground thyme

- 1 teaspoon ground white pepper

- ½ teaspoon garlic powder

- ½ teaspoon ground black pepper

- 1 whole whole chicken

Directions:

1. Mix salt, paprika, cayenne pepper, onion powder, thyme, white pepper, garlic powder, and black pepper together in a small bowl.
2. Rub seasoning mixture over the entire chicken to evenly season.
3. Put rubbed chicken into a large resealable plastic bag refrigerate 8 hours to overnight.
4. Remove chicken from bag and cook in slow cooker on Low until no longer pink at the bone and the juices run clear, 4 to 8 hours.
5. An instantread thermometer inserted into the thickest part of the thigh, near the bone should read 165 degrees F 74 degrees C.

Pan Seared Shrimp & Browned Zucchini Salad

Ingredients:

- 1/2 tsp olive oil

- 10 shrimps peeled, keep the ends

- pinch of salt

- 3/4 cup arugula salad

- 1/3 cup + 1/3 cup water

- 1 cup chopped yellow zucchini

For the salad dressing:

- 1/2 lemon juiced

- 1 oz 30 g fatfree Greek yogurt

- 1 tsp mustard

- 1 tsp warm water

- 1/4 tsp salt

- 1 sachet sweetener

Directions:

1. Combine ingredients for salad dressing in a bowl and whisk until wellmixed.
2. Pour 1/3 cup of water into a large nonstick skillet, then add in chopped zucchini.
3. Cook the zucchini with water over medium heat, until water, has evaporated and zucchini lightly stick to the pan, stirring occasionally.
4. Add in more water about 1/3 cup and repeat the same until the zucchini is browned to your liking. Add the browned zucchini to the salad dressing.
5. Preheat olive oil in a nonstick skillet.

6. Lightly coat the shrimps with salt, then cook in a single layer until turned pink.

7. Turn the shrimps and continue cooking until just cooked through.

8. Add the shrimp and arugula to the zucchini and toss to mix well.

Salmon And Broccoli Tabbouleh

Ingredients:

- Small handful parsley, chopped

- Small handful mint, chopped 2 spring onions, trimmed and sliced

- Grated zest of ½ lime

- 1 salmon fillet

- Seasoning salt and pepper to taste

- 2 tablespoons oat bran

- 1/3 cup broccoli florets

Directions:

1. Place the oat bran in a bowl and pour over 2 tablespoons boiling water and leave to stand for 10 minutes.

2. Sream or blanch the broccoli in boiling water then refresh under cold running water. fluff the oat bran with a fork then stir in the chopped herbs, spring onion, lime zest, broccoll and seasoning.

3. Grill the salmon fillet to your liking and serve with the tabbouleh.

4. Alternatively you could flake the fish and stir into the tabbouleh to serve.

Stuffed Baked Tomatoes

Ingredients:

- 7 ounces extralean ham, finely chopped

- 2 tablespoons very finely chopped fresh basil

- 8 tomatoes

- Salt and freshly ground black pepper

- 4 eggs

Directions:

1. Preheat oven to 425°F.
2. Cut the tops off the tomatoes spoon out the insides, sprinkle a little salt inside, and turn them over on a plate to let their juices drain.

3. In a medium bowl, beat the eggs, season with salt and pepper to taste, and add the ham and basil.
4. Turn the tomatoes over and place them in a baking dish. Spoon the egg mixture into the tomatoes and bake for 25 minutes.

Eggplant Frittata

Ingredients:

- 3 eggs

- 1 cup fatfree milk

- A pinch of ground nutmeg

- 3 sprigs of fresh thyme, chopped

- 3 sprigs of fresh rosemary, chopped

- 14 ounces eggplant, peeled and cut into ½inch slices

- Salt and freshly ground black pepper

- ⅛ Teaspoon vegetable oil

Directions:

1. Preheat oven to 300°F.
2. Place the eggplant slices in a colander, sprinkle them with a little salt and set them aside until their juices drain out, about 30 minutes.
3. Wipe the slices dry with a clean kitchen towel.
4. Bring a medium pot of water to a boil and blanch the eggplant for 5 minutes, then drain
5. In a medium bowl, mix the eggs, milk, nutmeg, thyme, rosemary, and salt and pepper to taste until thoroughly combined.
6. Coat a 9 × 9inch baking dish with the oil and wipe out any excess with a paper towel.
7. Arrange the eggplant slices in the prepared baking dish and pour the egg mixture over the eggplant.
8. Bake for 30 minutes.

Omelets With Anchovy Sauce

Ingredients:

- 2 tablespoons fatfree milk

- 10 fresh chives, finely chopped

- 5 sprigs of fresh cilantro, finely chopped

- 5 sprigs of fresh parsley, finely chopped

- Salt and freshly ground black pepper

- ⅜ teaspoon vegetable oil, divided

- 6 sundried tomatoes, rehydrated and chopped

- 3 tomatoes, stems removed and quartered

- 8 canned anchovies, rinsed, dried, and chopped

- 1 tablespoon capers, drained and rinsed

- 8 eggs

Directions:

1. Heat a nonstick skillet over medium heat.
2. Add ⅛ teaspoon of the oil and wipe out any excess with a paper towel. Add the tomatoes, anchovies, and capers.
3. Cook, stirring often, for 5 minutes.
4. Transfer the sauce to a small bowl and set aside.
5. In a medium bowl, beat together the eggs, milk, chives, cilantro, and parsley, plus salt and pepper to taste.
6. Reheat the skillet over medium heat, coat with ⅛ teaspoon of the oil, and wipe out any excess with a paper towel.

7. Pour in half the egg mixture and cook the eggs until set, about 10 minutes.

8. Transfer the omelet to a plate. Repeat with the remaining oil and the rest of the egg mixture.

9. Let the omelets cool, then cut them into strips ¾ inch wide.

10. Place the omelet strips in a shallow bowl, add the sauce and the sundried tomatoes, and gently toss until well combined. Serve warm.

Ovenbaked Salmon

Ingredients:

- 2 lemon slices per serving

- Freshly ground black pepper, to taste

- 1 salmon fillet per serving

Directions:

1. Preheat your oven to 450 F.
2. Place a piece of aluminum foil on your work surface, shiny side up.
3. Place 2 lemon slices on the foil and place the salmon fillet on top of the lemon slices. Season fillet with pepper.
4. Fold the foil loosely into a sealed packet around the fillet, allowing room for heat to expand the packet as it steams.

5. Bake for 1822 minutes until the fish is cooked, opaque, and flakes easily with a fork.

Thai Chicken Patties

Ingredients:

For chicken patties

- Fresh coriander 2 tbsp

- 1 green chili, roughly chopped

- ½ Red onion, chopped

- 1clove garlic, chopped

- 1 small fresh ginger, peeled and chopped

- Ground chicken 350 gm

For dip

- Greek yogurt 250 gm

- Chopped fresh chives 2 tbsp

- Pepper and salt to taste

- 3 spring onions, chopped

- A splash of lemon juice

Directions:

1. For making dip, blend all the Ingredients: together in a food processor until smooth.
2. Shift to the bowl, flavor to taste with pepper and salt.
3. Cover the bowl and chill in the refrigerator.
4. For making Thai patties, mix all the Ingredients: except ground chicken in a blender and blend.
5. Mix ground chicken and the mixture thoroughly and then mould six small cakes using your hands.

6. Grease nonstick pan and place on the stove over medium high heat.
7. Add patties and cook for about 10 minutes until golden brown.
8. Serve with dip.

Lemon Chicken

Ingredients:

For marinade

- 1 cube of fresh sliced ginger

- Juice of one lemon

- 1 red chili, chopped

- 1 whole Chicken, chopped

- A handful of fresh chopped coriander

- 1 large garlic clove, sliced

For dip

- Chopped fresh parsley 2 tbsp

- Pepper and salt to taste

- Chopped fresh chives 2 tbsp

- Paprika ½ tsp

- Fatfree Greek yogurt 250 gm

Directions:

1. For marinade, Mix all the Ingredients: except Chicken together in bowl.
2. Take chopped chicken in a separate bowl and add marinate.
3. Stir well and place in the refrigerator for about an hour.
4. Now for dip, mix all the Ingredients: together in a bowl and flavor it with pepper and salt.
5. Chill in the refrigerator until the chicken is done.

6. Remove chicken from marinate and cook in the oven for about 25 minutes until golden brown.
7. Serve with dip.

Grilled Halibut Fillets

Ingredients:

- 1 teaspoon salt

- 1 teaspoon ground black pepper

- 1 tablespoon fresh lemon juice

- 1 tablespoon chopped fresh parsley

- 2 6 ounce halibut fillets

- 1 clove garlic, minced

- 6 tablespoons olive oil

- 1 teaspoon dried basil

Directions:

1. Mix together all the spices in a bowl with the lemon juice and olive oil.
2. Add in the halibut fillets. Combine all Ingredients: thoroughly to allow the spices to seep into the fillet.
3. Put the mixture inside a resealable bag. Seal it, and then massage the fillet again.
4. Marinate the fish with the mixture for about an hour by storing it in the refrigerator.
5. Once your grill has been preheated, take the marinated fish fillet out of the refrigerator, and drain the excess marinade.
6. Grill over open flame for about five minutes.
7. Remove from grill, serve, and enjoy.

Bread Crumbcheese Coated Chicken Breast

Ingredients:

- 1 cup dry bread crumbs

- 2/3 cup grated Parmesan cheese

- 1 teaspoon dried basil leaves

- ¼ teaspoon ground black pepper

- 2 tablespoons olive oil

- 1 clove garlic, minced

- 6 skinless, boneless chicken breast halves

Directions:

1. For baking the mixture, grease a baking dish 9x13 inches in dimension, and preheat the oven to 350 degrees F 175 degrees C.
2. In separate bowls, make the oil and bread crumb mixture.
3. The oil mixture consists of a combination of olive oil and garlic.
4. For the bread crumb mixture, combine the bread crumbs, cheese, basil leaves, and pepper.
5. Coat each chicken with oil mixture, first followed by the bread crumb mixture.
6. Align the coated chicken on the pregreased baking dish. Sprinkle the remaining bread crumbs on the chicken.
7. Bake for 30 minutes.
8. Let cool for a bit, around ten minutes before serving.

Black Eye Peas With Greens

Ingredients:

- 3 cloves garlic minced

- 1 carrot peeled and diced

- 1 cup red bell pepper diced

- 1/2 teaspoon smoky paprika or liquid smoke

- 1 tsp dried oregano

- 1/2 teaspoon dried thyme

- 1/2 teaspoon sea salt

- 1 pound dry black eyed peas

- 1 cup yellow onion diced

- 1/4 teaspoon freshly ground black pepper

- 6 cups lowsodium vegetable broth

- 2 cups chard spinach or collard greens, sliced optional

Directions:

1. Rinse peas under running water and remove any bad peas and small stones.
2. Transfer to a medium saucepan. Cover in water by at least 3 inches and soak for at least 6 hours to overnight. Drain and rinse beans under cold water.
3. To a large pot over medium heat add 1/4 cup water or vegetable broth, diced onion, garlic, carrots, and bell pepper.
4. Sauté, stirring occasionally, until the onions are translucent.
5. Add liquid smoke, oregano, salt, and pepper. Sauté a few more minutes.

6. Add drained beans and vegetable broth.

7. Bring to a boil, reduce heat, and simmer, covered, about 45 minutes or until beans are tender. Add more broth as necessary.

8. Stir in chard and simmer another 5 minutes until wilted. Season with salt and pepper.

Date Paste

Ingredients:

- 2 cups water

- 4 cups pitted dates

Directions:

1. Cover dates with boiling water and allow to sit for at least 30 minutes.
2. Drain reserving 2 cups of the soaking water.
3. In a highpowered blender, blend dates and the soaking water on high for a few minutes until it becomes a paste. Add more water if it's difficult to blend or too thick
4. Store paste in a covered glass jar and refrigerate for up to 3 months or longer.

Warm roasted red pepper and cauliflower pate

ingredients:

- 1 tsp. cumin

- ¼ roasted red pepper

- 1 garlic clove

- 1 whole cauliflower

- ½ c. skim milk

Directions:

1. Boil cauliflower in saucepan with water for 25 min. Drain well.
2. Pour all the Ingredients: into a blender and blitz until wellcombined.

3. Pour the milk slowly into the blender until desired consistency is reached. Serve warm.

Aromatic Roasted Roots

Ingredients:

- 1 celeriac

- 1 bulb garlic, halved

- 5 parsnips

- 5 carrots

- ½ swede rutabaga

Directions:

1. Preheat oven to 350°F.

   Peel and cut all carrots and parsnips into quarters.

2. Peel the celeriac and swede, and cut them into 1inch cubes.

3. Use an oil spray or 12 drops of oil inside a roasting pan to prevent the vegetables from sticking to pan.

4. Place garlic and vegetables into pan. Roast for about 5060 minutes or until the vegetables are tender.

Ovenroasted Turkey

Ingredients:

- Salt and pepper to taste

- 35 medium size shallots

- 2 tbsp. dried sage

- 1 whole turkey

- 1 tbsp. ground cumin

- 2 tbsp. dried sage

- Olive oil cooking spray

Directions:

1. Preheat oven to 375°F.

2. Combine ground salt & pepper, ground cumin, dried thyme & sage.

3. Rub the spices gently into the bird. You can use the cooking spray to oil the skin.

4. Cut shallots into quarters. Place turkey inside of a roasting pan.

5. Place the shallots with the turkey inside a roasting bag.

6. Add 1 tbsp. of water. Using the bad allows you to use less fat to cook, thus saving on calories.

7. Cook time depends on size of turkey. About 2030min before the cooking time is up, cut open the roasting bag and let the brown a bit.

8. At this time, check to see how much longer the turkey needs to cook.

Creamy Lemon Cod

Ingredients:

- 4 tbsp. lemon juice

- Salt and dark pepper

- 1 cod filet

- 5 shallots, finely slashed 2 oz. sans fat
  fromage frais

- 1 ½ tbsp. mustard

Directions:

1. Preheat broiler to 350°F.
2. Place the shallots in warmed a pan with a
   sprinkle of water and decrease until it shallots
   relax and become clear.

3. Combine as one the fromage frais with the mustard, lemon squeeze, salt, and pepper.
4. Mix in shallots to cheddar combination.
5. Place the cod in a baking dish and pour the fromage frais over the fish. Heat in the broiler for 20 minutes.

Fluffy Dessert Meringues

Ingredients:

- 1 egg white

- 2 tablespoons of sweetener

Directions:

1. Preheat stove to 250°F.
2. Separate the white of egg into bowl. Dispose of yolk.
3. Beat the egg white with a hand or tabletop blender until tops structure.
4. Add sugar to bowl and keep blending until joined.
5. Spoon enormous scoopfuls onto baking plate fixed with material paper.
6. Permit to heat for 45 minutes or until they dry and solidify.

7. Allow meringues to cool totally prior to eliminating from baking tray.
8. Serve finished off with organic product, cream, or pudding.